The Spanish Flu

Detailed History of The Great Influenza of 1918. Global Consequences, Historical Analysis and Lessons that Humanity Have Learned from The Deadliest Plague

---

Robert Aceveds

© **Copyright 2020 by Robert Aceveds**
All rights reserved.

This document is geared towards providing exact and reliable information with regard to the topic and issue covered. The publication is sold with the idea that the publisher is not required to render accounting, officially permitted, or otherwise qualified services. If advice is necessary, legal or professional, a practiced individual in the profession should be ordered.

From a Declaration of Principles which was accepted and approved equally by a Committee of the American Bar Association and a Committee of Publishers and Associations.

In no way is it legal to reproduce, duplicate, or transmit any part of this document in either electronic means or in printed format. Recording of this publication is strictly prohibited and any storage of this document is not allowed unless with written permission from the publisher. All rights reserved.

The information provided herein is stated to be truthful and consistent, in that any liability, in terms of inattention or otherwise, by any usage or abuse of any policies, processes, or directions contained within is the solitary and utter responsibility of the recipient reader. Under no circumstances will any legal responsibility or blame be held against the publisher for any reparation, damages, or monetary loss due to the information herein, either directly or indirectly.

Respective authors own all copyrights not held by the publisher.

The information herein is offered for informational purposes solely and is universal as so. The presentation of the information is without a contract or any type of guarantee assurance.

The trademarks that are used are without any consent, and the publication of the trademark is without permission or backing by the trademark owner. All trademarks and brands within this book are for clarifying purposes only and are owned by the owners themselves, not affiliated with this document.

Table of Contents

INTRODUCTION..2

CHAPTER 1 6

HISTORY 6

CHAPTER 2 28

EXAMPLES ON HOW PANDEMICS HAVE CHANGED HUMAN HISTORY.......................28

CHAPTER 3 67

ORIGINS OF THE PANDEMIC OF 1918..........67

CHAPTER 4 83

GLOBAL EFFECTS OF THE DEADLIEST PLAGUE IN HISTORY 83

CHAPTER 5 96

HOW THE USA REACTED TO THE CRISIS ..96

CHAPTER 6 107

LESSONS TO REMEMBER FROM THE GREAT INFLUENZA 1918 -1920.....................107

CHAPTER 7 111

SIMILARITIES AND COMPARISON WITH
THE ACTUAL WORLD PANDEMIC 111

CONCLUSION...117

Robert Aceveds

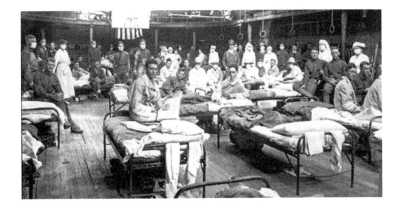

INTRODUCTION

The Spanish flu was a deadly influenza pandemic caused by the H1N1 influenza A virus, also known as the 1918 flu pandemic. It infected 500 million people – around a third of the world's population at the time – in four consecutive waves from February 1918 to April 1920. Usually, the death toll is believed to have been anywhere between 17 and 50 million, making it one of the most deadly pandemics in human history.

In the USA (in Fort Riley, Kansas, Haskell County, and in New York City), France (Brest), the United Kingdom, and Germany, the first reports of disease and mortality were recorded. World War I censors suppressed these early reports to maintain morale. Newspapers were free to portray the consequences of the epidemic in neutral Spain, such as King Alfonso XIII's grave illness. Those reports gave Spain a false impression of being extremely hard hit. This brought about the name "Spanish flu." Historical and epidemiological evidence is insufficient to establish the pandemic's geographic origin with certainty, with differing views as to its place.

Most influenza diseases kill the very young and the very old overwhelmingly, with a higher survival rate for those in between. However, The Spanish flu pandemic has resulted in a higher than expected mortality rate for young adults. Scientists give some potential reasons for the high mortality rate of the 1918 influenza pandemic. Some analyzes have shown that the virus is especially deadly because it causes a cytokine storm that ravages young adults' stronger immune systems. In comparison, a 2007 review of medical journals from the pandemic era showed that the viral infection was no more aggressive than previous influenza strains. Instead, malnutrition, overcrowded medical camps, and hospitals revealed that the virus was no more aggressive than previous influenza strains. Most victims were killed by this superinfection, usually after a very prolonged death bed.

The Spanish flu of 1918 was the first of two pandemics caused by the influenza A virus H1N1; the second was the swine flu pandemic of 2009.

While its geographical origin is uncertain, the disease was called Spanish flu from the pandemic's first wave. Spain was not active in the war, remained neutral, and had not enforced wartime censorship. Consequently, newspapers were free to report the consequences of the outbreak, such as King Alfonso XIII's serious illness, and these widely circulated reports created a false impression.

At the time of the pandemic, alternative names were also used. Similar to The Spanish flu name, many of these even pointed to the disease's supposed roots. In Senegal, it was named 'the Brazilian flu,' and in Brazil, it was named 'the German flu,' while in Poland, it was known as 'the Bolshevik disease. In Spain itself, the flu nickname, the 'Naples Soldier,' was adopted from an operetta in 1916, The Song of Forgetting (La canción del olvido), after one of the librettists whipped that the most famous musical number of the play, Naples Soldier, was as catchy as the flu.

Other names for this virus include the "1918 influenza pandemic," the "1918 flu pandemic".

CHAPTER 1

HISTORY

The first wave of early 1918

The pandemic is historically identified as having started on March 4, 1918, with the report of Albert Gitchell, an army cook at Camp Funston in Kansas, USA, despite the possible incidence of cases before him. The disease was observed in Haskell County in January 1918, causing local doctor Loring Miner to alert the academic journal of the US Public Health Service.

As the US entered World War I, the disease spread rapidly from Camp Funston, a major training ground for American Expeditionary Forces soldiers, to other US Army camps and Europe, becoming an outbreak in the Midwest,

East Coast, and French ports by April 1918, and reaching the Western Front by mid-month.

The first flu outbreak lasted from the first quarter of 1918 and was comparatively mild. Mortality rates were not significantly higher than normal; in the United States, ~75,000 flu-related deaths were registered in the first six months of 1918, compared to ~63,000 deaths in 1915 during the same period. In Madrid 1918, fewer than 1,000 people died from influenza between May and June. However, the first wave triggered a massive interruption to World War I military operations, with three-quarters of French troops, half of the British forces, and over 900,000 wounded German soldiers.

The Spanish Flu

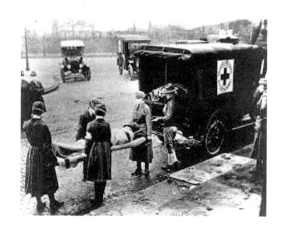

The deadly second wave of late 1918

This wave began in the second half of August, possibly traveling by ships from Brest to Boston and Freetown, Sierra Leone, where it had originally arrived for naval training with American troops or French recruits. From the Camp Devens and Boston Navy Yard, about 30 kilometers west of Boston, other US military sites were soon affected, as were troops being transported.

From Europe, the second wave passed across Russia on a diagonal South-West-Northeast direction. As well as being carried to Arkhangelsk by the intervention of North Russia, and then spread across Asia after the Russian Civil War and the Trans-Siberian railway, reaching Iran (where it spread through the Holy City of Mashhad), and later India in September, as well as Japan and China in October.

The pandemic of 1918's second wave was even more lethal than the first. The first outbreak had resembled traditional flu epidemics; the sick and the aged were the most at risk, while younger, healthy people quickly recovered. October 1918 was the month with the greatest death rate of the entire pandemic. Between September-December 1918, ~292,000 deaths were reported in the US, compared to ~26,000 in the same timeframe in 1915. Copenhagen recorded more than 60,000 deaths, Holland estimated more than 40,000 deaths from influenza and acute respiratory diseases, and Bombay recorded ~15,000 deaths in a population of 1: m

The third wave of 1919

The third wave of Spanish flu reached Australia in January 1919, killing 12,000 after lifting a maritime quarantine. Then, it spread rapidly across Europe and the United States, where it continued through the spring and until June 1919. It mainly affected Spain, Serbia, Mexico, and Great Britain, leading to hundreds of thousands of deaths. In the United States, sporadic outbreaks occurred in several cities like Los Angeles, New York City, San Francisco, St. Louis, Memphis, and Nashville. In the first six months of 1919, total American mortality rates were in the tens of thousands.

The fourth wave of 1920

In spring 1920, a fourth wave erupted in isolated areas, including New York City, Scandinavia, Switzerland, and several South American islands. New York City alone recorded 6,374 deaths between December 1919 and April 1920, nearly twice the first wave in spring 1918. Other US cities, including Kansas City, Minneapolis, Detroit, Milwaukee, and St. Louis, were hit particularly hard.

Potential origins

Despite its name, historical and epidemiological evidence are unable to establish The Spanish flu's geographical origin. However, several theories were suggested.

United States of America

The first confirmed cases occurred in the US. In 2003, historian Alfred W. Crosby claimed that the flu originated in Kansas, and the famous author John M. Barry identified an outbreak in Haskell County, Kansas, in January 1918 as the point of origin in his 2004 article.

A 2018 study of tissue slides and medical records performed by evolutionary biology professor Michael Worobey found evidence against Kansas-born disease as these cases were milder and had fewer deaths compared to New York City infections over the same time. Via phylogenetic analysis found evidence that the virus was possible of North American origin, but it was not definitive. Moreover, the virus' haemagglutinin glycoproteins indicate that it originated well before 1918, and other findings show that the reassortment of the H1N1 virus was possibly taking place in or around 1915.

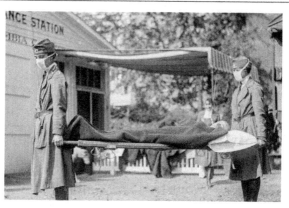

Europe

Virologist John Oxford has theorized the main UK troop staging and hospital camp in Étaples in France as being at the core of Spanish flu. His research found that in late 1916 the Etaples camp was struck by the emergence of a new high-mortality disease that caused symptoms similar to flu. According to Oxford, a similar epidemic occurred in March 1917 at the army barracks in Austria. Thousands of victims of gas attacks and other war injuries were treated at the hospital, and every day 100,000 soldiers passed the camp. It was also the home of a piggery, and poultry was frequently brought in to feed the camp from nearby villages. Oxford and his colleagues postulated that a bird-harbored precursor virus mutated and spread to pigs near the front.

A study released in 2016 in the Journal of the Chinese Medical Association discovered proof that the 1918 virus circulated in the European armies for months and probably years before the 1918 pandemic. Details from the Austrian archives were released by political scientist Andrew Price-Smith, indicating that it started in Austria in early 1917.

China

In 1993, Claude Hannoun, the Pasteur Institute's leading expert on flu in 1918, reported that the precursor virus was likely to have originated from China and then evolved in the United States near Boston, spreading to Brest, France, the battlefields of Europe, the rest of Europe, and the rest of the world, with sailors and allied soldiers as the main spreaders. Humphries, of Newfoundland Memorial University in St. John's, based his observations on newly discovered documents. He found archival evidence that a respiratory disease that affected northern China (where the laborers came from) in November 1917 was reported as similar to Spanish flu by Chinese health officials a year later. However, no tissue samples have survived for modern comparison. However, some records of respiratory disease were on parts of the track that the laborers took to get across.

One of the few parts of the world that seemed to be less affected by the flu pandemic of 1918 was China. Many studies recorded a relatively mild flu season in 1918 (although this is contested for lack of data during the War period, see Around the Globe). This led to the hypothesis that the flu pandemic of 1918 occurred in China since the lower rates of flu mortality can be explained by the Chinese population's previously established immunity to the flu virus.

A report published in the Journal of the Chinese Medical Association found no evidence that the 1918 virus was introduced into Europe via Chinese and Southeast Asian soldiers and workers. Instead, it found evidence of its spread in Europe before the pandemic. The 2016 study indicated that the low flu mortality rate among the Chinese and Southeast Asian workers in Europe meant that the 1918 influenza pandemic couldn't have originated there. Further proof against the disease being spread by Chinese workers was that workers entered Europe through other routes that didn't result in a detectable spread, making them unlikely to have been the original hosts.

Transmission and mutation

The basic reproductive number of the virus ranged between 2 and 3. World War I close quarters and large troop movements hastened the pandemic, and all undoubtedly increased transmission and increased mutation. Also, the war may have decreased the resistance of people to the virus. Some believe that the immune systems of soldiers have been compromised by malnutrition and the pressures of war and chemical attacks, which have increased their susceptibility. Increased travel was a significant factor in the worldwide incidence of the flu. Modern transport networks made it easier for troops, sailors, and civilian travelers to spread the disease. Another factor was government deception and denial, leaving the populace ill-prepared to cope with the outbreaks.

The magnitude of the second wave has been attributed to the circumstances of World War I. Natural selection favored a moderate strain in civilian life. Many that get very sick remain at home, and those who are slightly sick resume their lives, spreading the slight burden preferentially. Natural selection was inversed in the trenches. Soldiers with a mild strain remained where they were, and the seriously ill were sent to crowded field hospitals on packed ships, spreading the deadlier virus. The second wave started, and the flu rapidly spread all over the world. Therefore, during modern pandemics, health workers looked for deadlier strains of a virus as it entered social upheaval areas. The fact that most of those who have recovered from first-wave outbreaks have become resistant has proven that it may have been the same strain of flu. This was most vividly demonstrated in Copenhagen, which survived with a total death rate of just 0.29 percent (0.02 percent in the first wave and 0.27 percent in the second wave) due to exposure to the first less-lethal wave. The second wave was much more dangerous for most of the population; the most vulnerable were those like the soldiers in the trenches – adults who were young and fit.

New cases suddenly dropped after the deadly second wave struck in late 1918. For example, in Philadelphia, 4,597 people died in the week ending October 16, but influenza had almost vanished from the city by November 11. One reason for the gradual decrease in the disease's lethality is that the doctors have become more effective in preventing and treating pneumonia formed after the patients have contracted the virus. In his 2004 book The Great Influenza: The Epic Story of the Deadliest Plague In History, John Barry claimed that researchers find no evidence to support this position. Another hypothesis holds that the 1918 virus evolved extremely rapidly to a lower lethal form. Such influenza evolution is common: pathogenic viruses appear to become less lethal over time, as hosts of more deadly strains begin to die out. Some fatal cases continued until March

1919, killing one player in the 1919 Stanley Cup Finals.

Symptoms and Signs

The majority of those infected suffered only the usual flu symptoms of sore throat, headache, and fever, particularly during the first wave. However, the illness was far more serious during the second wave, frequently aggravated by bacterial pneumonia, which was sometimes the cause of death. This more severe form would contribute to the development of heliotropic cyanosis, whereby the skin would first develop two mahogany spots over the cheekbones, which would then spread to color the entire face blue, followed by black coloration first in the extremities and then further spreading to the limbs and the torso. After this, death would follow within a few hours or days because of the lungs being filled with fluids. Other symptoms and signs reported included spontaneous mouth and nosebleeds, miscarriages for pregnant women, a peculiar smell, hair falling, delirium, dizziness, insomnia, loss of hearing or smell, and blurred and impaired color vision. An observer wrote: "One of the most striking of the complications was hemorrhage from mucous membranes, especially from the stomach, intestine, and nose. Bleeding from the ears and petechial hemorrhages in the skin also occurred". The intensity of the symptoms was believed to be caused by cytokine storms (a physiological reaction in humans in which innate immune system causes an uncontrolled release of pro-inflammatory molecules named cytokines).

Most deaths have been from bacterial pneumonia, a common influenza-related secondary infection. This pneumonia was itself triggered by widespread upper respiratory tract bacteria, which could get into the lungs through the victims' infected bronchial tubes. The virus also killed people by causing major hemorrhages and edema in the lungs. Modern research has shown that the virus is especially deadly because it causes a cytokine storm (overreaction of immune symptoms in the body). During a cytokine storm, the animals experienced increasingly progressive respiratory failure and death. Young adults' strong immune reactions were asserted to have destroyed the body, while children and middle-aged adults' weaker immune reactions resulted in fewer deaths among those categories.

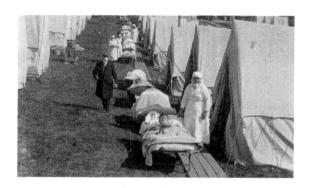

Misdiagnosis

Since the virus that triggered the disease was too small to be seen under a microscope at the time, there were issues with a proper diagnosis. Instead, the bacterium Haemophilus influenzae was incorrectly believed to be the cause, as it was big enough to be seen and was present in many, but not all patients.

During the deadly second wave, there were also concerns that it was probably influenza, dengue fever, or cholera. Another common misdiagnosis was typhus, prevalent in social upheaval circumstances, which subsequently also afflicted Russia in the aftermath of the October Revolution. In Chile, the country's elite view was that the nation was in extreme decline, and therefore the presumption was that the nation was in serious deterioration.

Public health management

Although there were mechanisms for alerting public health authorities to infectious spread in 1918, they usually did not include influenza, which resulted in a slow response. Nevertheless, the action was taken. Maritime quarantines have been imposed on islands such as Iceland, Australia, and American Samoa, saving many lives. Social distancing steps have been adopted, such as closing classrooms, theaters, and places of worship, limiting public transport, and banning mass gatherings. Face masks have become widespread in some countries, such as Japan, although there have been concerns about their effectiveness. Vaccines were also created, but because they were focused on bacteria and not on the actual virus, they could only help with secondary infections. Various restrictions were eventually enforced.

A later study showed that interventions such as banning mass meetings and requiring face mask wear could reduce death rates by as much as 50 percent, but this depended on them being introduced early in the outbreak and not removed prematurely.

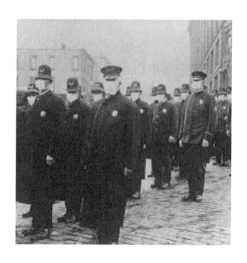

Medical treatment

Since there were no antiviral drugs to treat the virus and no antibiotics to treat secondary bacterial infections, doctors would rely on a random variety of medicines of varying degrees of efficacy, such as aspirin, digitalis, strychnine, Epsom salts, quinine, arsenic, castor oil, and iodine. Herbal medicine treatments, such as bloodletting, Ayurveda, and Kampo, were also used to treat the flu.

Information dissemination

Because of World War I, many countries participated in wartime censorship and censored pandemic reporting. For instance, the Italian newspaper Corriere della Sera was forbidden from publishing regular death tolls. The newspapers of the time were also largely paternalistic and concerned about mass panic. Misinformation would also spread along with the epidemic. In Ireland, there was a belief that noxious gases had emerged from the mass graves of Flanders Fields and were "blown by winds all over the world. "It was often suspected that the Germans were behind it, for example, by poisoning the aspirin created by Bayer or by releasing poison gas from U-boats.

Around the globe

The Spanish flu has infected about 500 million people, approximately one-third of the world's population. It is estimated that the number of infected people who died varies widely, but flu is known as one of the most deadly pandemics in history. It is estimated from 1991 that between 25 and 39 million people died from the virus. A 2005 report placed the death toll at 50 million (approximately 3 million citizens).

Let's see how many people were murdered by the disease in many parts of the world. Approximately 12-17 million people died in India, about 5 percent of the population. The death toll in the British-ruled districts of India was 13.88 million. Another estimate suggests at least 12 million deaths. The decade between 1911 and 1921 was the only census period in which India's population dropped, mainly because of the destruction of The Spanish flu pandemic.

Twenty thuosand died out of 210,000 infected in Finland. In Sweden, 34,000 died.

Twenty-three million people were affected in Japan, with at least 390,000 deaths reported. In the Netherlands East Indies (now Indonesia), 1.5 million were believed to have died among 30 million inhabitants. In Tahiti, 13 percent of the population died during a month. Similarly, 22 percent of the population (38,000) in Western Samoa died within two months.

In New Zealand, an estimated 6,400 Pakeha and 2,500 indigenous Maori were killed by the flu in six weeks, with Maori dying eight times Pakeha's rate.

In the United States, about 28% of the 105 million people were contaminated, and 500,000 to 850,000 died (0.48 to 0.81% of the population). Native American tribes were especially hard hit. There were 3,293 recorded deaths among indigenous Americans in the region of the Four Corners. Entire Inuit and Alaskan indigenous village populations died in Alaska. Fifty thousand died in Canada.

Three hundred thousand have died in Brazil, including president Rodrigues Alves.

As many as 250,000 died in Britain, more than 400,000 in France.

In Ghana, the influenza outbreak killed at least a hundred thousand people. Tafari Makonnen (Emperor of Ethiopia, the future Haile Selassie) was one of the first Ethiopians to contract The Spanish flu yet survive. Many of his subjects did not; figures for deaths ranged from 5,000 to 10,000 or higher in the capital city of Addis Ababa.

Russia's death toll was estimated at 450,000, but the epidemiologists who proposed this figure called it a "shot in the dark." If it is right, Russia lost approximately 0.4 percent of its population, which means it experienced the lowest influenza-related mortality in Europe. Another study finds this figure impossible, considering that the country was in the midst of civil war and the everyday life system had broken down; the study indicates that Russia's death toll was closer to 2 percent or 2,7 million people.

Robert Aceveds

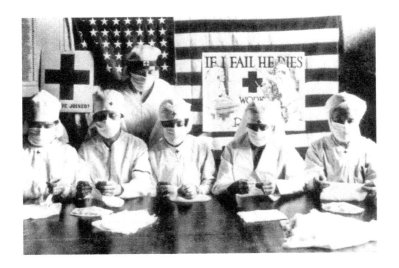

CHAPTER 2

EXAMPLES ON HOW PANDEMICS HAVE CHANGED HUMAN HISTORY

Pandemics have had a significant impact throughout history in influencing human society and politics. They have caused the fall of empires from the Justinian Plague of the sixth century to The Spanish flu of the last century, weakened pre-eminent forces and governments, generated social unrest, and brought down wars. Here's a summary of some of the deadliest pandemics and how they affected human history.

THE JUSTINIANIC PLAGUE

In the sixth century, one of the deadliest pandemics in documented history broke out in Egypt and spread quickly to Constantinople, the capital of the Eastern Roman (Byzantine) Empire.

The plague took its name from the then Byzantine Emperor Justinian. The disease, spreading from Constantinople to both East and West, had killed as many as 25 to 100 million people. The plague struck Constantinople when the Byzantine Empire, under Justinian's rule, was at the height of its power. Most of the traditionally Roman Mediterranean coast had been invaded by the Empire, including Italy, Rome, and North Africa.

The plague would return in various waves, ultimately disappearing in AD 750, after dramatically weakening the Empire. As the Byzantine Army struggled to hire new soldiers and maintain military supplies to battlegrounds, their provinces were under attack amid the disease's outbreak. Constantinople had also been hit hard economically by the plague, greatly weakening its war machine. The Empire had lost lands in Europe to the Germanic-speaking Franks and Egypt, and Syria to the Arabs by the time plague vanished.

Plague Origination & Transmission

Originating in China and Northeastern India, the plague (Yersinia pestis) was transported to

Africa's Great Lakes area through overland and sea-trade routes. Egypt was the starting point for the Justinianic Plague. The Byzantine historian Procopius of Caesarea (500-565 CE) described the plague's beginning on the Nile River's northern and eastern shores at Pelusium. The virus spread in two directions, according to American author Wendy Orent: North to Alexandria and East to Palestine.

The black rat (Rattus rattus) was the means of transmission of the plague, which traveled on the grain ships and carts sent as a tribute to Constantinople. North Africa was the principal source of grain for the Empire in the 8th century and various goods, including paper, ivory, oil, and slaves. The grain was stored in large warehouses, so it provided the fleas and rats with the ideal breeding ground, essential for plague transmission.

In Justinian's Flea, William Rosen argues that while rats are known to eat just about anything (including vegetable and small animals), the grain is their favorite meal. Rosen further notes that rats do not usually move more than 200 meters from their birthplaces during their lifespan. While on the grain boats and carts, however, the rats were borne all over the country.

According to historian Colin Barras, during the time, Procopius reported the climatic changes taking place in southern Italy: unusual snow and frost incidents in mid-summer, lower average temperatures, and more equatorial sunshine. So a decades-long cold snap started with social disturbances, war, and the first known plague outbreak. The colder than average weather affected crop harvests, resulting in food shortages that led to people moving across the country. These hesitant migrants had been followed by plague-infected, flea-ridden rats. The ideal conditions for an outbreak were created by cold, exhausted, hungry people on the go, coupled with illness and disease in the middle of warfare and a growing population of rats carrying a highly contagious disease. And what an outbreak it would be: named after the Byzantine emperor Justinian I (482-565 CE), the plague has infected almost half of Europe's population.

Types Of Plague & Symptoms

Based on DNA analysis of bones found in graves, the kind of plague that struck the Byzantine Empire during Justinian's reign was bubonic (Yersinia pestis). However, the other two plague types, pneumonic and septicemic, were also very likely present. It was also the bubonic plague that would devastate Europe in the 14th century (better known as the Black Death), killing more than 50 million people, or almost half of the continent's entire population. And in Justinian's time, the plague was not new to history. Author Wendy Orent argues that the first known account of bubonic plague is revealed in the Old Testament, in the tale of the Philistines who stole the Israelites' Ark of Covenant and succumbed to "swellings."

In Secret History, Procopius describes patients as suffering from visions, dreams, fevers, and swellings in the neck, armpits, and behind their ears. Procopius relates that although some patients have fallen into comas, some have been profoundly psychotic. Some of the patients suffered for days before death, while others died almost instantly after symptoms started. The explanation of Procopius's disease almost definitely indicates the existence of bubonic plague as the principal culprit of the epidemic. He blamed the Emperor for the outbreak, declaring Justinian either a ghost or that the Emperor was being punished by God for his evil ways.

How the plague spread through the Byzantine Empire?

War and trading encouraged the spread of the disease throughout the Byzantine Empire. Justinian spent the early years of his rule battling several enemies

- fighting for control of Italy by Ostrogoths;
- fighting for power against Vandals and Berbers in North Africa;
- fending off Franks, Slavs, Avars, and other primitive tribes engaged in attacks against the Empire.

Historians also indicated that for the rats and fleas carrying the plague, soldiers and the supply trains assisting their war activities served as transmission means. By 542 CE, Justinian had reconquered much of his kingdom, but, as Wendy Orent points out, stability, prosperity, and trade had provided enough conditions to encourage an outbreak of plague. Constantinople, the Eastern Roman Empire's administrative capital, served as the Empire's commercial commerce center. The positioning of the capital along the Black and Aegean Seas has made it the ideal crossroads for commercial routes from China, the Middle East, and North Africa. Where commerce and trade went, so went fleas, rats, and the plague.

The disease path is chronicled by author Wendy Orent. The plague spread from Ethiopia to Egypt, and then throughout the Mediterranean region, following the Empire's developed trade routes. Neither Northern Europe nor the countryside transmitted the disease, indicating that the black rat was the infected flea's primary carrier, as the rats held close to the ports and ships. The outbreak in Constantinople lasted about four months but would last for approximately the next three centuries, with the last epidemic registered at 750 CE. No further large-scale outbreaks of plague will arise before the episode of the Black Death in the 14th century.

The plague was so prevalent that no one was safe; the epidemic also affected the Emperor, but he did not die. Dead bodies littered the streets of the capital. Justinian directed troops to help clear the bodies. When the graveyards and tombs had been filled, burial pits and trenches had been dug to accommodate the surge of dead people. In homes, corpses were disposed of, dumped into the sea, and loaded on boats for seaside burials. And it was not just human beings who were affected: animals of all sorts, including cats and dogs, died and needed proper disposal.

Plague Treatment

People who had been infected had two courses of action: medical care or home remedies. William Rosen describes the medical staff as being mainly qualified doctors. Many doctors took part in a four-year research course taught by professional teachers of medicine- the iastrophists, at Alexandria, then at the leading medical training center. The students' education focused primarily on the Greek physician Galen (129-217 CE), who was inspired by the philosophy of humorism in his interpretation of the disease. This medical method depended on the treatment of body fluid-based illness, known as "humor."

Due to lack of access to one of the types of doctors - court, private, public - people often turned to home remedies. Rosen describes numerous methods that people have taken to cure the plague, including cold-water baths, saint-blessed powders, magic amulets & rings, and various medications, especially alkaloids. Failing all primary care methods, people either went to hospitals or were subject to quarantine. According to Rosen, the survivors were credited with "good fortune, sound underlying health, and an uncompromising immune system."

Effects on the Byzantine Empire

The plague episode led to a political and economic collapse of the Byzantine empire. As the disease spread across the Mediterranean world, it undermined the Empire's ability to fight its enemies. By 568 CE, Northern Italy was effectively conquered by the Lombards and defeated the tiny Byzantine garrison, leading to the fragmentation of the Italian peninsula, which remained split and divided until re-unification in the 19th century. The Empire was unable to stop the encroachment of Arabs in the Roman provinces of North Africa and the Near East.

The decreased size, and the Byzantine Army's inability to combat outside forces, was mainly due to its failure to attract and train recruits because of the spread of disease and death. The demographic decline not only affected the military and the defenses of the Empire, but the Empire's economic and administrative systems started to crumble or vanish.

Trade was interrupted in the Empire. The agricultural sector, in particular, had been destroyed. Fewer people meant fewer farmers were growing less food, which caused prices to soar and tax revenues to fall. The near-collapse of the economic system did not dissuade Justinian from demanding his demoted people the same amount of taxes. The Emperor proceeded to wage wars against the Goths in Italy and the Vandals at Carthage, in his attempt to restore the former dominance of the Roman Empire, lest his rule disintegrate. Even the Emperor remained committed to several public works and church building projects in the capital, including the Hagia Sophia building.

In his Secret History, Procopius recorded almost 10,000 deaths that afflicted Constantinople every day. Modern historians who predicted 5,000 deaths a day in the capital city have doubted his precision. However, 20-40 percent of Constantinople's inhabitants will ultimately die of the disease. Nearly 25 percent of the population died in the remainder of the Empire, with figures ranging from 25 to 50 million people.

THE BLACK DEATH

The most deadly pandemic recorded in human history has been the Black Death, or pestilence, that hit Europe and Asia in the 14th century.

According to various figures, it killed between 75 to 200 million people. The plague had reached China, India, Syria, and Egypt in the early 1340s. It arrived in Europe in 1347, where the disease killed up to 50 percent of the population. The epidemic has also had lasting social and economic effects.

As Stanford historian Walter Scheidel puts it, pandemics are one of the "four horsemen" that have flattened injustice. The remaining three are wars, revolutions, and failures by the state. Mr. Scheidel writes in his book, The Great Leveler, how the Black Death led to better wages for serfs and farm laborers. "The world became more prosperous with labor (after the death of millions of workers). Soil rents and interest rates fell. Landowners stood to lose, and employees could expect to make a profit." he writes. Wages in parts of Europe tripled as demand for labor increased. And as the economy began to change, the landowning class forced authorities to monitor the increasing labor cost. In England, the Crown passed legislation in this regard, establishing the tensions from which the Peasant Rebellion of 1381 would inevitably arise. The pandemic has also contributed to the systematic persecution of the Jews in Europe. In several parts of the continent, Jews, blamed for spreading the disease, were burned alive.

The Black Death's most important influence may have been the deterioration of the Catholic Church. As Frank M. Snowden, a Yale professor and author of Epidemics and Culture, observed: from the Black Death to the present, the pandemics outbreak questioned the relationship between man and God. "How could it be that such an occurrence could take place with a wise, omniscient, all-knowing divinity? " In a recent interview, he said: The Church was as powerless as any other institution as the plague spread throughout the continent like wildfire, which shook the people's confidence in the Church and the clergy. While the Church would remain as a powerful institution, before the outbreak of the plague, it would never recover the strength and prestige it had enjoyed. In the 16th century, the Protestant Reformation will further undermine the Catholic Church.

How Did The Black Plague Start?

Even before the "death ships" pulled to port at Messina, many Europeans had heard reports of a "Great Pestilence" carving a deadly path through Near and Far East trade routes. The epidemic had also reached China, India, Persia, Syria, and Egypt in the early 1340s.

The plague is believed to have arisen in Asia more than 2,000 years ago and was possibly transmitted by trading ships. However, recent research has shown that the Black Death's pathogen may have existed in Europe as early as 3000 BC.

Symptoms of the Black Plague

Europeans were scarcely prepared for Black Death's terrifying truth. "In both men and women," wrote the Italian poet, Giovanni Boccaccio, "at the beginning of the epidemic, some swellings, either on the groin or under the axes ... waxed to the bigness of a common apple, others to the size of an egg, some more and some less, and these the vulgar named plague-boils."

Blood and pus sprang from these odd swellings, accompanied by a host of other nasty symptoms-vomiting, diarrhea, terrible aches, fever, chills, and pains, and then death.

The Bubonic Plague affects the lymphatic system, causing lymph nodes to swell. The infection will spread to the blood or the lungs if untreated.

How Did The Black Death Spread?

The Black Death was terrifyingly, indiscriminately contagious: "the mere touch of the skin," Boccaccio wrote, "appeared to itself to transmit the disease to the toucher." People who were perfectly safe at night when they went to bed could be dead by morning.

Did you know? Many scholars claim the "Ring around the Rosie" nursery rhyme was written about the signs of Black Death.

Understanding the Black Death

Today, scientists recognize that a bacillus called Yersinia pestis spread the Black Death, also known as the plague. (In the late 19th century,

French biologist Alexandre Yersin discovered the germ.)

They know the bacillus spreads through the air from person to person, and even through infected fleas and rats. Almost everywhere in medieval Europe, both of these pests could be found, but they were especially at onboard home ships of all kinds — which is how the dreaded plague made its way through one European port city after another.

Not long after Messina was struck, the Black Death spread to France's Marseilles port and North Africa's Tunis harbor. Then it entered two cities in Rome and Florence, in the middle of a complex network of trade routes. The Black Death had reached Paris, Bordeaux, Lyon, and London by mid-1348.

Today this horrific series of events is tragic but understandable. However, there seemed to be no reasonable reason for it in the middle of the 14th century.

Nobody knew exactly how the Black Death was transmitted from one patient to another, and nobody knew how to avoid it or handle it. For example, according to one doctor, "instant death happens when the aerial spirit that escapes from the sick man's eyes reaches the healthy person standing nearby and looking at the ill."

How Do You Treat the Black Death?

Physicians relied on primitive and unsophisticated methods such as bloodletting and boil-lancing (practices that were both risky and unsanitary) and superstitious practices such as rosewater or vinegar burning medicinal herbs and bathing.

In the meantime, healthy people in a panic have done whatever they could to stop the sick. Doctors declined to see patients, priests denied last rites, and shopkeepers shut down their shops. Many people fled to the countryside from the towns, but they were unable to avoid the disease even there: it infected cows, horses, goats, pigs, and chickens as well as humans.

So many sheep died that a European wool shortage was one of the results of the Black Death. Many people, struggling to save themselves, have even given up their loved ones, sick and dying.

"Therefore," Boccaccio wrote, "everybody thought of gaining immunity for themselves."

Black Plague: God's Punishment?

Since they did not understand the nature of the disease, many people assumed that the Black Death was a form of divine punishment - retribution for crimes against God, such as greed, fornication, blasphemy, or heresy worldliness.

By this reasoning, the only way to surmount the plague was to obtain forgiveness from Heaven. Some people thought the way to do this was to rid their cultures from heretics and other troublemakers - so in 1348 and 1349, for example, several thousands of Jews were massacred. (Thousands more fled to Eastern Europe's sparsely populated regions where they could be relatively protected from the rampaging crowds in the cities.)

Some coped with the Black Death epidemic's fear and confusion by lashing out at their neighbors; others coped by turning inward and fretting over their soul's state.

Flagellants

Some upper-class men joined flagellant processions that traveled from town to town and participated in public shows of penance and punishment: they would beat each other with thick leather belts filled with sharp metal parts while the townspeople looked on. The flagellants repeated the procedure three times a day for 33 1/2 days. They'd then move on to the next town and start the process over again.

While the flagellant movement brought some consolation to people who felt impotent in the face of unexplained disaster, the Pope, whose authority the flagellants had started to usurp, soon began to worry. The revolution had disintegrated in the face of this papal opposition.

How Did The Black Death End?

The epidemic never really stopped, and it returned years later with a vengeance. But officials in Ragusa's Venetian-controlled port city were able to slow their spread by keeping sailors in isolation until it was clear they didn't carry the disease -

creating social distancing that depended on isolation slow disease spread.

The sailors were initially held for thirty days (a Trentino) on their ships, which later increased to 40 days, or a quarantine - the root of the word "quarantine" and a still used procedure today.

Does The Black Plague Still Exist?

The outbreak of Black Death had run its course by the early 1350s, but the disease reappeared for centuries every few years. Current sanitation and public-health policies have significantly mitigated but have not removed the effects of the disease. According to the World Health Organization, while antibiotics are available to treat Black Death, there are only 1,000 to 3,000 plague cases per year.

THE SPANISH FLU

The Spanish flu, which broke out during the last quarter of the First World War, was the most devastating pandemic of the past century that killed as many as 50 million. First, the flu was reported in Europe and then spread rapidly to

America and Asia. India, one of the hardest affected by the pandemic, has lost 17 to 18 million people, around 6 percent of its population.

The outbreak had one of the big impacts on the outcome of the battle. While the flu reached both sides, the Germans and Austrians were so severely impacted that their offensives were derailed by the outbreak. In his book, My War Memoirs, 1914-18, German general Erich Ludendorff wrote that flu was one reason for Germany's loss. In March 1918, Germany launched its Spring Offensive on the west front. The disease had debilitated the German units by June and July. "Our Army was hurting. Influenza was rampant. In its aftermath, it always left a bigger vulnerability than the doctors knew, "he wrote. On November 11, 1918, the Armistice was signed, which ended the war. Yet the flu will keep ravaging areas of the world for several months to come.

What Is the Flu?

Flu or influenza is a virus that attacks the breathing system. The flu virus is highly contagious: breathing droplets are produced and spread into the air when an infected individual coughs, sneezes, or speaks, and can then be inhaled by everyone nearby.

Also, someone who touches something with the virus on it and then touches their mouth, nose, or eyes can become infected with it.

Did you know? During the 1918 flu epidemic, the health commissioner in New York City attempted to slow down the flu spread by forcing businesses to open and close staggered shifts to prevent overcrowding on the subways.

Every year, flu outbreaks occur and differ in magnitude depending partly on what form of the virus is circulating. (The flu viruses can mutate rapidly.)

Flu Season

"Flu season" in the US normally runs from late fall through spring. More than 200,000 Americans are treated for flu-related complications in a single year. According to CDCP (the Centers for Disease Control and Prevention), there have been about

3,000 to 49,000 flu-related US deaths annually in the last three decades.

Young children, people over the age of 65, pregnant women, and people with some medical conditions, such as asthma, diabetes, or heart disease, face an elevated risk of flu-related complications, including influenza, ear or sinus infections, or bronchitis, among others.

A flu pandemic such as that of 1918 happens when a highly virulent new influenza virus appears for little to no immunity and spreads rapidly across the globe, from person to person.

Spanish Flu Symptoms

The 1918 pandemic's first wave emerged in the spring and was usually mild. The sick, who had such common flu symptoms as chills, fever, and exhaustion, generally recovered after a few days, and the number of deaths reported was minimal.

In the fall of the same year, a second extremely infectious outbreak of influenza emerged with a vengeance. Victims died within a few hours or days of developing symptoms, turning their skin blue and filling their lungs with fluid, which caused them to suffocate. In one year only, in 1918, America's average life expectancy plunged by a dozen years.

What Caused The Spanish flu?

Where exactly the particular strain of influenza that caused the pandemic emerged is unknown; however, the flu of 1918 was first observed in Europe, America, and Asia before spreading to virtually every other region of the world within a matter of months.

Although the flu of 1918 was not localized from one region, it became known worldwide as The Spanish flu, since Spain was hit hard by the disease and was not subject to the blackouts of wartime news that plagued other European countries. (Alfonso XIII, king of Spain, allegedly contracted the flu.)

One peculiar feature of the 1918 flu was that it struck down several relatively healthy youths. This community is usually immune to this infectious disease, including several servants from World War I.

The Spanish Flu

The 1918 flu caused more US soldiers to die than they were killed in combat during the war. Around 40% The US Navy was struck with the flu, while 36 percent of the army became sick, and soldiers in crowded ships and trains traveling across the world helped spread the killer virus.

While the death toll due to The Spanish flu is mostly estimated at 20 million to 50 million victims worldwide, other figures are as high as 100 million victims - about 3% of the world's population. The numbers are impossible to know due to a lack of medical record-keeping in many places.

But what is known is that few areas were immune to the flu of 1918 - in America, casualties ranged from inhabitants of major cities to rural villages in Alaska. In early 1919, also President Woodrow Wilson allegedly contracted the flu while negotiating the Treaty of Versailles, which ended World War I.

Why Was it Called The Spanish flu?

The Spanish flu did not occur in Spain, while the Spanish press was the only one to report it.

During World War I, Spain was a neutral country with a free media covering the outbreak from the beginning, first writing on it in Madrid late May 1918. Meanwhile, there were wartime censors from Allied countries and Central Powers who covered up flu reports to keep morale up. Since Spanish news sources were the only ones reporting on the flu, many assumed that it originated there (the Spanish, meanwhile, claimed that the virus came from France and called it the "French Flu").

Where Did The Spanish flu Come From?

Scientists still don't know for sure where The Spanish flu came from, but hypotheses point to France, China, Britain, or the United States, where the first confirmed case was registered on March 11, 1918, at Camp Funston in Fort Riley, Kansas.

Some assume infected soldiers spread the disease around the country to other military bases and took it overseas. 84,000 American soldiers marched through the Atlantic in March 1918, and a further 118,000 were followed the next month.

Fighting The Spanish flu

When the flu struck in 1918, physicians and scientists were confused about what caused it, or how it was treated. Unlike today, there were no reliable vaccines or antivirals, the flu-treating medications. (In the 1940s, the first approved flu vaccine appeared in America. Over the next decade, vaccine manufacturers could regularly develop vaccines that would help contain future pandemics.)

Complicating matters was that parts of America had been left with a shortage of doctors and other health workers in World War I, and many of the medical professionals available in the USA came down with the flu itself.

Additionally, in some areas, hospitals were so overwhelmed with flu patients that schools, private homes, and other buildings had to be converted into temporary hospitals, some of which were staffed by medical students.

Officials placed quarantines in certain areas, requiring residents to wear masks and close down public locations, including classrooms, churches, and theatres. People were told not to shake hands and remain indoors, libraries stopped lending books, and spitting prohibition laws were passed.

According to The New York Times, boy Scouts in New York City approached people they'd seen vomiting on the street during the pandemic and gave them cards that read: "You're in breach of the Sanitary Code."

The flu has a massive impact on society

The flu took on a substantial human toll, wiping out whole families and leaving numerous widows and orphans in its wake. Funeral parlors were overloaded and lined up corpses. Many people have had to dig graves for family members of their own.

The Spanish flu also has been harmful to the economy. Businesses were forced to shut down in the United States because too many of the workers were sick. Because of the flu-stricken population, essential services such as mail delivery and garbage collection were disrupted.

There weren't enough farmworkers in some areas to harvest crops. Both state and local health departments closed for service, hampering attempts to chronicle the flu outbreak in 1918 and provide answers to it to the public.

How the US Cities Tried to Stop the 1918 Flu Pandemic

In the summer of 1918, a devastating second wave of Spanish flu reached the American shores. Returning troops infected with the disease spread it to the general population - especially in densely populated cities. It fell to local mayors and healthy officials without vaccination or approved treatment plan to improvise measures to safeguard the welfare of their residents. Many made poor choices, with pressure to appear patriotic at wartime and a distorted media downplaying the spread of the disease.

The reaction from Philadelphia has been too little, too late. Dr. Wilmer Krusen, the city's director of public health and charities, insisted that mounting deaths were not due to The Spanish flu, but to the usual flu. Thus the city moved ahead on

September 28 with a Liberty Loan parade attended by tens of thousands of Philadelphians, spreading the disease like wildfire. About 1,000 Philadelphians were dead in just ten days, with another 200,000 sick. Only then did saloons and theaters closed in the whole town. By March 1919, more than 15,000 Philadelphia residents had lost their lives.

St. Louis, Missouri, was different: closed schools and cinemas, and prohibited public meetings. The peak mortality rate in St. Louis was thus just 1-8 of the death rate in Philadelphia at the pandemic period.

Citizens of San Francisco were fined $5 -a large amount at the time - if they were found without masks of public and charged with disrupting the peace.

Spanish Flu Pandemic Ends

The Spanish flu pandemic ended by the summer of 1919 when those infected either died or developed an immunity.

Nearly 90 years later, researchers revealed in 2008 that they had discovered what made the flu so lethal in 1918: a group of three genes made it possible for the virus to damage the bronchial tubes and lungs of a victim, and also paved the way for bacterial pneumonia.

Many other influenza pandemics have occurred since 1918, but none were as deadly. A flu pandemic from 1957 to 1958 killed about 2 million people worldwide, including about 70,000 in the US, and a pandemic from 1968 to 1969 killed around 1 million people, including about 34,000 Americans.

About 12,000 Americans died during the 2009-2010 H1N1 (or "swine flu") pandemic. The novel epidemic of 2020 is spreading across the world as countries scramble to find a cure for SARS-CoV-2 and people shelter in closed places to prevent the disease from spreading, which is especially deadly since many carriers are asymptomatic for days before they know they are infected.

Each of these modern-day pandemics is bringing renewed concern and attention to The

Spanish flu, or the so-called "forgotten pandemic," because its spread has been overshadowed by WWI's deadliness and covered up by news blackouts and inadequate record keeping.

THE ASIAN INFLUENZA

In 1957, another flu pandemic, also known as the Asian flu of 1957 or Asian flu pandemic of 1957, was first detected in East Asia in February 1957 and then spread to countries worldwide. The flu pandemic of 1957 was the second major influenza pandemic to occur in the 20th century; it followed the 1918–19 influenza pandemic and preceded the flu pandemic of 1968. The flu epidemic in 1957 caused an estimated one to two million deaths worldwide and is widely considered the least severe of the three 20th century influenza pandemics.

The outbreak in 1957 was caused by a virus known as Influenza A virus subtype H2N2 (A/H2N2). Analysis has shown this virus to be a reassorting strain (mixed species) from avian influenza strains and human influenza viruses. In

The Spanish Flu

the 1960s, several minor genetic changes were made to the human H2N2 strain, a phenomenon known as antigenic drift. These minor improvements carried with them occasional epidemics. After ten years of evolution, the flu virus of 1957 vanished, having been replaced by a new influenza A subtype, H3N2, which gave rise to the 1968 flu pandemic by antigenic change.

The virus spread across China and its neighboring regions during the first months of the flu pandemic of 1957. It had entered the United States by mid-summer, where very few people seem to have initially been affected. However, several infection cases were recorded several months later, especially in young children, the elderly, and pregnant women. This upsurge resulted from a second pandemic disease outbreak that hit the Northern Hemisphere in November 1957. The pandemic was already prevalent in the UK at that time as well. In England and Wales, a total of about 3,550 deaths had been recorded by December. The second wave was especially destructive, and the United States had suffered an estimated 69,800 deaths by March 1958.

Asian Flu Symptoms

Asian flu results in similar symptoms to many other influenza strains, including chills, cough, weakness, fever, body aches, and appetite loss. Influenza virus causes many of the symptoms widely reported in Asian Flu. Influenza is a respiratory disorder, so dry cough, sore throat, and breathing problems are all commonly documented among those suffering from the flu. Influenza typically leads to high fever and chills or body aches. A person can have no appetite and lose weight afterward. It can take several weeks to recover from H2N2; complications include pneumonia, strokes, heart failure, and death.

Asian Flu Deaths

The Asian Flu virus was first discovered in Guizhou. In February 1957, it spread to Singapore, reached Hong Kong by April, and reached the US by June. The death toll was around 69,800 in the United States. The elderly were particularly vulnerable. Worldwide death figures differ greatly depending on the source, varying from 1 million to

4 million, with "only two million" being settled by the WHO.

The epidemic of 1957 was related to the flu pandemic of 1968, by variance in severity and course of illness. Although some infected people had only moderate symptoms, such as cough and mild fever, others experienced life-threatening complications such as pneumonia. Many individuals unaffected by the virus were thought to possess defensive antibodies to other, closely related influenza strains. The rapid production of a vaccine against the H2N2 virus and the availability of antibiotics to treat secondary infections have restricted the pandemic's spread and mortality.

HUMAN IMMUNODEFICIENCY VIRUS

HIV is a virus that resides in blood, sexual fluids, and breast milk in humans. It weakens your immune system, so your body fights hard against common germs, viruses, fungi, and other invaders. It spreads primarily through unprotected sexual contact and needle-sharing.

AIDS is the disease that occurs when the immune system stops working, and you get sick because of HIV.

Who Gets It?

The infection spreads from individual to individual when there is an exchange of such body fluids, usually during vaginal or anal intercourse, or injecting drugs. Tattoos and body piercing may also be spread from rusty needles. It can be transmitted by oral sex, but the chance is small.

When the baby is exposed to its mother's infected blood during childbirth, or to her breast milk, a mother can transfer HIV to her infant. But in some developing world areas, breastfeeding for a mother with HIV is safer than giving a newborn formula with potentially contaminated water, especially if she receives HIV treatment.

HIV does not exist in saliva, tears, urine, or sweat - so it can not spread with these body fluids through casual touch.

HIV is not as readily obtainable as other infectious diseases. The virus can not live outside of the human body for long; it easily dies when it dries up. It is not propagated by livestock or insects. It won't be seen on public surfaces such as door handles or toilet seats.

HIV test is carried out on all blood products used in the United States and Western Europe today. Blood banks are getting rid of any blood donated that tests positive, so they never get into the public supply. Anyone who donates HIV-positive blood will be called so their doctor can examine them, and they will not be able to give blood again.

Where Is It Widespread?

HIV is spread worldwide, but Sub-Saharan Africa (the Southern part) has the largest number of people infected. The World Health Organization and UNAIDS office report that over one-third of adults are infected with HIV in certain parts of Africa. Many cases of HIV occur in South and Southeast Asia. In Eastern Europe, the number of people living with HIV is rising due to injection drug use.

The virus has two major types: HIV-1 and HIV-2. HIV-2 is most often present in West Africa, although it is also seen in other parts of the world. Tests for HIV usually look for both forms.

Living With HIV and AIDS

In the United States, the first known AIDS case was in 1981 (retrospectively, some cases had occurred earlier in the world). Since then, about 35 million people have died in the world from disease-related illnesses. Because of this, millions of children were orphaned.

Now, integrated drug therapies have turned HIV into a long-term infection you can handle, even though HIV has advanced toward AIDS. At the end of 2017, about 37 million people lived with HIV in the world, including around 2 million children. Of these individuals, about 22 million received these life-saving treatments. You will live a long time and have a near-average life expectancy if you work closely with your doctors and stick to your treatment plan.

It may take several years for HIV to weaken your immune system enough to make you vulnerable to certain diseases, such as a type of skin cancer called Kaposi's sarcoma. Many other "opportunistic diseases" are indicators of you getting AIDS, since people with strong immune systems never get them. If started early, the HIV treatments will prevent progression to AIDS.

Since there are medications that you can take for it, certain groups of people feel they no longer need to worry about HIV, while they are more likely to get the virus. But therapies don't alter the fact that HIV is a life-threatening disease.

Medicines for HIV and AIDS may be demanding. Despite successful initiatives in resource-limited countries to treat people with HIV, many people worldwide living with the virus and its complications still have trouble accessing the treatment they need.

CHAPTER 3

ORIGINS OF THE PANDEMIC OF 1918

The influenza pandemic of 1918–1919 infected more people than any other epidemic outbreak in human history. The lowest death toll estimate is 21 million, although the latest reports showed between 50 and 100 million deaths. The world population then was just 28 percent of what it is now, and most deaths happened in a period of sixteen weeks, from mid-September to mid-December 1918.

But it was never clear where this pandemic originated. Since influenza is an infectious disease, not necessarily an epidemic disease, this question can not be answered with utter certainty. Nonetheless, a British scientist has undertaken a comprehensive review of current medical and lay literature looking for epidemiological evidence in seven years of work on a pandemic history – the only evidence accessible. The analysis indicates the most probable place of origin in January 1918 was Haskell County, Kansas, a rural and sparsely populated county in the state's southwest corner. If this theory is right, it would have consequences for public policy.

But it is important to study other theories of the site of origin before providing the proof for Haskell County. Some epidemiologists and medical historians have theorized that the pandemic started in Asia in 1918, citing a deadly pulmonary disease outbreak in China due to the pandemic. Others also suggested that the virus was transmitted by either Chinese or Vietnamese workers crossing the USA or employed in France.

British scientist J.S. Oxford has speculated that the pandemic of 1918 began in a post of the British Army in France wherein 1916, an epidemic of British doctors called "purulent bronchitis" erupted. Autopsy records of soldiers killed by this epidemic – we can today label the cause of death as ARDS (acute respiratory distress syndrome) – bear a striking resemblance to those killed by influenza in 1918.

Yet, there are issues with certain alternative theories. Numerous investigators looked for the origins of the epidemic during the pandemic of 1918–1919. The American Medical Association funded what is widely considered the best out of the extensive international pandemic studies undertaken by the editor of The Journal of Infectious Disease, Dr. Edwin Jordan. He spent years analyzing facts worldwide; his thesis was published by the American Medical Association in 1927.

Since many influenza pandemics were already well-known in preceding centuries and had originated from the East, Dr. Jordan first considered Asia to be the source. But they didn't find any proof. Influenza emerged in China at the beginning of 1918, but the outbreaks were small and did not spread.

Contemporary Chinese scientists, educated by researchers from the Rockefeller Institute for

Medical Research (now Rockefeller University), reported that they assumed these outbreaks were infectious diseases unrelated to the pandemic. Jordan also looked at the deadly pulmonary disease described as influenza by some scholars, but this has been identified as a pneumonic plague by contemporary scientists. By 1918 the plague bacillus could be detected reliably and conclusively in the laboratory. So after monitoring all reported respiratory disease outbreaks in China, Jordan concluded that none of them "could be considered the true precursor" of the pandemic.

Jordan also took Oxford's theory to cause the "purulent bronchitis" in British Army camps in 1916 and 1917. He denied it on many grounds. True, the disease had flared up, but had not spread quickly or widely beyond the infected bases; it seemed to disappear instead. Since we now know a mutation can account for a virulent flare-up in an active influenza virus. For example, in the summer of 2002, an influenza outbreak exploded in Madagascar parts with incredibly high mortality and morbidity; in some towns, an absolute majority - in one instance, 67% of the population was sickened. But the virus that caused this outbreak was an H3N2 virus that would usually cause mild illness. Only 13 of 111 Health Districts in Madagascar were affected by the epidemic before it faded. There could have been something similar happening in the British base.

Jordan was exploring other potential pandemic sources in France and India in early 1918. He concluded that it was unlikely that either of them would trigger the pandemic.

That leaves the USA. There, Jordan observed a series of spring outbreaks. The proof appeared far clearer. One could see influenza jumping from Army camp to camp, then into cities, and heading to Europe. His conclusion: the place of origin was the United States.

A subsequent almost systematic, multi-volume British pandemic analysis agreed with Jordan. It also found no evidence of influenza sources in the Orient. It also dismissed the epidemic among British troops in 1916, and it also concluded: "The disease was possibly transported from the United States to Europe."

Macfarlane Burnet, Australian Nobel laureate, spent much of his research career focusing on influenza and closely followed the pandemic. He, too, concluded that the evidence was "strongly persuasive" that the disease began in the United States and spread with "American troops landing in France."

Before dismissing the findings of these contemporary investigators who lived through the pandemic and researched it, one must note how many of them were good. They were really good.

The Rockefeller Institute alone included extraordinary people whose investigators were deeply involved in the crisis. By 1912, his head Simon Flexner - his brother wrote the "Flexner Report" revolutionizing American medical education - used the immune serum to reduce the mortality rate for meningococcal meningitis from over 80 percent to 18 percent; by comparison, a study found a 25 percent mortality rate for bacterial meningitis at Massachusetts General Hospital in the 1990s. Peyton Rous was awarded the 1966 Nobel Prize for his 1911 work at the institute; he was well ahead of the scientific consensus. By 1918 Oswald Avery and others had already developed an effective curative serum and a vaccine for the most dangerous pneumococcal pneumonia at Rockefeller Institute. Avery would spend the remainder of his career researching pneumonia, at least partially because of the pandemic. The work led directly to his discovery of the "transforming theory"-his discovery that the genetic code is carried by DNA.

It is difficult to ignore the investigators' observations of this quality. Jordan was of this quality.

More evidence against Oxford's theory comes from Dr. Jeffrey Taubenberger, famous for his work extracting samples from preserved tissue from the 1918 virus and sequencing its genome. Initially, based on a statistical analysis of the virus's rate of mutation, he assumed that it existed two or three years before the pandemic. But more studies persuaded him that, only a few months before the pandemic, the virus appeared (J

The Spanish Flu

Taubenberger's personal contact with the author, June 5, 2003).

If the contemporary observers were correct, if American troops were bringing the virus to Europe, where did it begin in the United States?

Both modern epidemiological research and lay pandemic background have established the first documented widespread influenza outbreak at Camp Funston, now Ft. Riley, located in Kansas. Yet there was one location where an influenza outbreak, which was previously unknown - and unprecedented - occurred.

Three hundred miles west of Funston lay Haskell County, Kansas. The scent of manure there signified civilization. People raised grain, poultry, livestock, and hogs. Sod-houses was so prevalent that even one of the few post offices in the town was located in one. The population was 1,720 in 1918, spread over 578 square kilometers. But rough and raw as life may be, science in the form of Dr. Loring Miner had entered the region. Enamored of ancient Greece – he reread the classics in Greek regularly - he epitomized

William Welch's claim that "the outcomes of medical education were better than the method." His son was also a doctor, educated in a completely scientific way, serving in the Boston Navy.

In late January and early February 1918, Miner was unexpectedly hit with an influenza outbreak, but influenza, unlike anything he had ever seen. Soon hundreds of his patients - the best, healthiest, most vigorous in the county - were struck down as unexpectedly as if fired. One patient then progressed toward pneumonia. Then another one. And they started dieting. Local paper Santa Fe Monitor, evidently worried about damaging morale during the war, initially said nothing about the deaths but recorded on the inside pages in February: "Mrs. Eva Van Alstine is sick with pneumonia. Her little son Roy is now able to get up. Ralph Lindeman is still very sick. Goldie Wolgehagen works in the Beeman store during her sister Eva's illness. Homer Moody has been reported quite sick. Ralph McConnell has been quite sick this week".

The Spanish Flu

The outbreak escalated. It then vanished as suddenly as it came. He continued to work for men and women. Children went back in school. And the war reclaimed its grip on the minds of the people.

However, the disorder did not slip out of Miner's mind. Influenza was not a reportable disease, nor was it a disease tracked by any state or federal public health agency. Even Miner regarded the disease as a dangerous manifestation that he warned national public health authorities about. Public Health Statistics (now Morbidity and Mortality Weekly Report), a weekly newspaper published by the US. Public Health Service issued his message to alert health officials to outbreaks of infectious diseases worldwide. This would be the only reference in that journal to influenza anywhere in the world during the first six months of 1918.

Historians and epidemiologists have most likely overlooked Haskell since his study was not released until April and pointed to deaths on March 30, following outbreaks of influenza elsewhere. The county had been influenza-free by then. Haskell County, Kansas, is the first known instance of such an unusual influenza epidemic anywhere in the world that a doctor warned public health officials. It remains the first recorded instance, which indicates that a new virus was violently adapting to man.

If the virus was not found in Haskell, there is no clear reason for how it came in there. There were no other reported outbreaks elsewhere in the United States. Anyone might have transmitted the disease to Haskell, and there were no reports of influenza outbreaks in either media or expressed anywhere else in the country in vital statistics. And unlike the epidemic in France in 1916, one can trace the virus's path from Haskell to the outside world with complete clarity.

All county Army staff reported for training to Funston. Friends and family had visited them at Funston. Soldiers came home on leave and then went back to Funston. In late February, "Many people around the country are suffering from la grippe or pneumonia" (Santa Fe Monitor, February 21, 1918). It also noted, "Dean Nilson

The Spanish Flu

shocked his mates by coming home from Camp Funston on a five-day furlough. Dean looks like soldier life agrees with him." Ernest Elliot left for Funston to visit his brother when his child fell ill. John Bottom departed for Funston on February 28. "We expect John would make an excellent soldier," the paper said (February 28, 1918, Santa Fe Monitor).

These men were subjected to influenza, and presumably, others unnamed by the paper, since they have landed in Funston between February 26 and March 2. The first soldier at the camp declared ill at sick call on March 4 with influenza. Average 56,222 troops were retained at the camp. More than eleven hundred people were sick enough to need hospitalization within three weeks, and thousands more needed care at infirmaries scattered across the base – the exact number was not reported.

Whether or not the Haskell virus has spread worldwide, the Funston explosion's timing strongly suggests Haskell's influenza epidemic. In the meantime, Funston fed a steady stream of men to other American locations and Europe, men whose business was killing. They'd be more professional at it than they ever thought.

Soldiers moved between Funston and the outside world without interruption, especially to other Army bases and France. Greenleaf and Camps Forrest in Georgia saw their first influenza cases on March 18, and twenty-four of the thirty-six major army camps experienced an influenza outbreak by the end of April. Thirty of the country's fifty biggest cities have reported an April increase in excess influenza and pneumonia mortality. While this spring wave was relatively mild - the second wave of killing hit in the fall - some alarming results remain. A subsequent army study said, "First reported at this time was fulminating pneumonia, with wet hemorrhagic lungs, fatal in 24 to 48 hours." (Pathology records suggest what we now call ARDS.) Early April saw the first recorded autopsy of an influenza victim in Chicago. "The lungs were full of hemorrhages," the pathologist observed. He considered this odd enough to ask the then-editor of The Journal of Infectious Diseases to "look at it as a new disease".

The Spanish Flu

In France, first, at Brest, the single largest disembarkation port for American troops, influenza was erupting by then. By then, as MacFarlane Burnet later said, "It is easy to observe the influenza tale at this time primarily in terms of the experiences of the army in America and Europe."

It certainly helps that the 1918 pandemic likely originated in the United States because it tells researchers where to look for a new virus. They have to look around everywhere.

Why the Name "Spanish Flu"?

The influenza pandemic of 1918 was not originating in Spain, as many people claimed.

Mother Nature unleashed the deadliest strain of influenza in human history in the Spring of 1918, just as the human-made horrors of World War I were slowly beginning to wind down. For the next 18 months, the virus affected as many as 40 percent of the world population. Of these, an estimated 20 to 50 million people perished - more than the approximately 17 million people killed during World War I. The effect of the pandemic spread from the USA and Europe to Greenland and the Pacific Islands. Its victims included President Thomas Woodrow Wilson's, who contracted it in early 1919 while negotiating the Versailles Treaty.

When the pandemic reached epic proportions in 1918, it became widely referred to in the United States and Europe as the "Spanish Flu," or the "Spanish Woman." Many thought this was because, on the Iberian Peninsula, the illness had arisen, but the nickname was simply a widespread misunderstanding.

Spain was one of only a few European countries to remain neutral during the First World War. Unlike in the nations of the Allied and Central Powers, where wartime censors filtered Spanish Flu news to avoid public hysteria, the Spanish media were free to cover it in gory detail. The sickness first made headlines in late May 1918 in Madrid, and attention only expanded after the Spanish King Alfonso XIII came down a week later with a nasty outbreak. Since nations experiencing a media blackout could read-only in-depth reports from Spanish news outlets, they automatically believed the country was the ground zero for the pandemic. Meanwhile, the Spaniards assumed the virus had spread from France to them, so they took to call it the "French Flu."

Although the "Spanish Flu" is unlikely to have originated in Spain, scientists are still unsure of its source. Britain, France, and China have all been proposed as the possible birthplace of the virus, as has the United States, where on March 11, 1918, the first recorded case was identified at a Kansas military base. Researchers have also carried out detailed work on pandemic victims' remains, but they have yet to find out why the virus that devastated the world in 1918 was so deadly.

CHAPTER 4

GLOBAL EFFECTS OF THE DEADLIEST PLAGUE IN HISTORY

The world has seen an extraordinary change in health in the last 150 years. The visualization shows that life expectancy in many nations, which calculates death's average age, has doubled from about 40 years or less to over 80 years. This was not only an accomplishment in some countries; life expectancy in all regions of the world has doubled.

What also stands out is how sudden and crippling adverse effects in life expectancy the pandemics turn out to be. The most notable is the massive, rapid drop in life expectancy in 1918, caused by an unusually deadly influenza pandemic known as The Spanish flu.

To understand why life expectancy so abruptly decreased, one needs to consider what it means. The term life expectancy, which is the precise name for this metric, refers to the number of years a person can expect to live. Statisticians look only at the mortality rate of a given year and then measure this snapshot of population health as the average death age of a hypothetical generation of people for whom the mortality trend of that year will remain constant over their entire lives. Life expectancy for time is an indicator of the longevity of the population in one year.

This outbreak of influenza was not confined to Spain. It did not even originate there (recent research indicates that the epidemic occurred in New York due to evidence of a virus pre-pandemic wave in that city).

But it was called as such because Spain was neutral in the First World War (1914-18), which meant reporting on the nature of the pandemic was open, while countries fighting sought to suppress information about how influenza affected their people to preserve dignity and not appear vulnerable in the enemy's eyes.

In the Northern Hemisphere, the influenza epidemic began in the spring of 1918. The virus soon spread and gradually entered all parts of the world: the outbreak developed into a pandemic.

In a much less connected world, in the middle of the Pacific Islands, the virus gradually entered incredibly remote areas such as the Alaskan wilderness and Samoa.

Although peak mortality was achieved in 1918, in late 1920, the pandemic did not end until two years later.

The Global Death Count of The Spanish Flu Today

We already know that the death toll of a normal flu season can help provide a background for the severity of the influenza pandemics. The latest figures for the total number of Spanish Influenza deaths are about 400,000 deaths a year. Paget et al. (2019) propose an average of 389,000, from 518,000.4 with an uncertainty level of 294,000.

The Spanish Flu

This means that The Spanish flu has been responsible for the death of 0.0052 percent of the world's population in recent years - one person out of 18,750. As compared to the low death count estimate of Spanish flu (17.4 million), this pandemic, more than a century ago, induced a death rate 182 times higher than today's baseline.

How many people died in The Spanish flu and other influenza pandemics?

So many research teams have been working on the task of reconstructing the pandemic's global health effects. These estimates now have a lot of uncertainty, and while the theoretical debates continue, the range of estimates allows us to understand the magnitude of the case.

The visualization here shows the available estimates from the various research publication discussed in the following.

David Patterson and Gerald F. Pyle (1991) reported that the pandemic killed between 24.7 and 39.3 million people.

Johnson and Mueller's widely cited report (2002) arrives at a much higher estimate of 50 million deaths worldwide. But the authors say that this may be undervalued and that the real death rate was as high as 100 million.

Peter Spreeuwenberg et al. (2018), a more recent review, concluded that earlier estimates were too high. They estimate their deaths at 17.4 million.

Global death rate

How do these figures correlate then with the size of the world's population? How large was the share who died in the pandemic?

According to figures, in 1918, the world population was 1.8 billion.

On this basis, Spreeuwenberg et al. 's low estimate of 17.4 million deaths (2018) indicates that Spanish flu killed almost 1 percent (0.95 percent) of the world's population.

If we depend on the estimate of 50 million deaths reported by Johnson and Mueller, this means that 2.7 percent of the world's population was killed by Spanish flu. If it were significantly higher than 100 million, the global death rate would have been 5.4%, as these writers say.

Over this period, the world population increased by about 13 million per year, indicating that The Spanish flu era was possibly the last time in history when the world population declined.

Other large influenza pandemics

The Spanish flu pandemic was the biggest but not the only major influenza pandemic of modern times. The Russian flu pandemic (1889-1890) is estimated to have killed 1 million people two decades before The Spanish flu.

Estimates for the "Asian Flu" death toll (1957-1958) range from 1.5 million to 4 million. Gatherer (2009) reported an estimated 1.5 million, while Michaelis et al. (2009) released an estimate of 2–4 million.

According to a WHO publication, the "Hong Kong Flu" (1968-1969) killed between 1 and 4 million people.

Michaelis et al. (2009) released a 1–2 million lower estimate.

The 1977-78 Russian flu pandemic was induced by the same H1N1 virus that gave rise to Spanish flu. Around 700,000 died worldwide, according to Michaelis et al. (2009).

Two things become apparent from this overview: influenza pandemics are not unusual, but the 1918 Spanish Flu was the most severe influenza pandemic in recorded history.

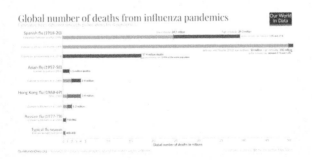

The effect of The Spanish flu pandemic on various age groups

Here this last graph demonstrates the life expectancy by age in England and Wales. The red line shows a newborn's life expectancy, with the rainbow-colored lines above illustrating how long a person can expect to live once they reach that specified older age. For instance, the light green line reflects life expectancy for children who had reached ten years of age.

It shows that life expectancy increased at all ages, indicating that the often-heard argument that life expectancy 'just' increased because decreasing infant mortality isn't valid. The emphasis of this accompanying text here is this long-term increase in life expectancy at all ages.

It is surprising and concerning that the effects of The Spanish flu that the illustration indicates how the pandemic had very little effect on older people. While life expectancy decreased by more than ten years at birth and young ages, there was no improvement in life expectancy among 60- and

70-year-olds. This contrasts with what we would expect: older populations seem to be more vulnerable to outbreaks of influenza and respiratory infections. Looking at today's mortality rates for lower respiratory infections (pneumonia) and upper respiratory infections, we can see that death rates are higher for people aged 70 and over.

One reason this pandemic was so destructive was that it accounted for a large proportion of the population among the young.

Why did older people become so immune to the pandemic of 1918?

The research literature indicates this was the case because older people had undergone an earlier flu epidemic – the already reported 'Russian flu pandemic' of 1889–90 - which provided some protection for the later Spanish Flu epidemic to those who lived through it.

The earlier pandemic of 1889-90 may have provided some immunity to the older population, but it was a devastating occurrence. One hundred thirty-two thousand people have died in England, Wales, and Ireland alone, according to Smith.

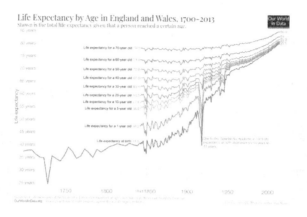

How The Spanish flu differs from the SARS-CoV-2 outbreak in 2020?

With all the writings of early March 2020, the question of how the current pandemic outbreak relates to The Spanish flu is a simple one. We have a study and data page dedicated to its outbreak.

There are several important variations which should be considered when contrasting today's pandemic with Spanish Flu:

1. They are not the same disease, and there are very different viruses that cause these diseases. The SARS-CoV-2-causing

virus is a virus from Coronaviridae family, not an influenza virus that caused The Spanish flu and the other influenza pandemics.

2. It seems the age-specific mortality is very different. As we've seen above, the 1918 Spanish Flu was extremely harmful to children and young people. Based on early reports in China, the latest virus causing SARS-CoV-2 seems most lethal to the elderly.

3. We've also seen above that several countries attempted to hide any information about influenza's epidemic during The Spanish flu. Data, analysis, and news sharing today are not perfect, but they are very different and far more accessible than in the past.

4. Today's world is indeed connected far better. It was railroads and steamships which connected the world in 1918. Aircraft today can transport humans and

viruses in a very short time to many corners of the globe.

5. Differences are also relevant in the health systems and infrastructure. In the days before antibiotics were developed, The Spanish flu reached the world, and many deaths, possibly the most, were not caused by the influenza virus, but by secondary bacterial infections. Morens et al. (2008) found that "most deaths ... likely resulted directly from secondary bacterial pneumonia caused by widespread upper respiratory tract bacteria" during The Spanish flu.

6. Not only health services were different but also the global population's health and living conditions. The 1918 pandemics affected a world population where a very large percentage was extremely poor-large proportions of the population were undernourished, people lived in very poor health in most parts of the world, and overcrowding, bad

sanitation, and low hygiene standards were common.

7. Also, a global war had devastated the populations in many parts of the world. Public resources were scarce, and many countries only invested huge portions of their money on the war.

Although much of the world is now much wealthier and healthier, the fear even today is that the SARS-CoV-2 epidemic will strike the poorest people the hardest.

These discrepancies mean one should be vigilant in drawing lessons from the outbreak a hundred years ago.

But The Spanish flu also reminds us how great a pandemic's effects can be, even in countries that have already been active in improving the population's health. A new pathogen can cause appalling destruction and lead to millions of deaths. That is why The Spanish flu has been cited as an alert and a reason to plan well for major pandemic outbreaks, which many researchers believed to accomplish.

CHAPTER 5

HOW THE USA REACTED TO THE CRISIS

The devastating second wave of Spanish flu arrived on America's shores in the late summer of 1918. Carried by doughboys returning home from Europe during World War I, the newly virulent virus first traveled from Boston to New York and Philadelphia before heading west to infect terrified communities from St. Louis to San Francisco.

Lack of a vaccine or even an established cause of the outbreak left to improvise to the mayors and town health officials. Will the schools be closed and all public hearings baned? Will every person need to wear a face mask with a gauze? Or would it be unpatriotic to close down essential financial hubs in times of war?

The Spanish flu killed an estimated 675,000 Americans and a whopping 20 to 50 million people worldwide when it was all over. Some US cities did much worse than others. Looking back, over a century later, we find evidence that the earliest and most well-organized responses delayed the spread of the disease- at least temporarily - while cities that lost their feet or let their guard down paid a heavier price.

By mid-September, The Spanish flu spread like wildfire through the Philadelphia army and naval facilities. Still, Wilmer Krusen, Philadelphia director of Public Health and Charities, told the public that the killed soldiers were suffering only from the old-fashioned seasonal flu and that it would be controlled before infecting civilians.

When the first few civilian cases were registered on September 21, local physicians worried that this could be the start of an outbreak, but Krusen and his medical board said that by staying warm, keeping their feet dry and their "bowels open," Philadelphians might lower their risk of catching the flu, writes John M. Barry in

The Great Influenza: The Story of the Deadliest Pandemic in History.

As the rates of civilian infections increased daily, Krusen declined to cancel the upcoming Liberty Loan parade scheduled for September 28. Barry writes that Krusen has been warned by infectious disease experts that the parade, expected to draw several hundred thousand Philadelphians, will be "a ready-made inflammable mass for a conflagration."

Krusen argued that the parade should proceed as it would collect millions of dollars in war bonds, and he played down the risk of the disease spreading. A patriotic parade of troops, marching bands, boy scouts, and local dignitaries marched 2 miles through downtown Philadelphia with spectator-packed sidewalks on September 28.

Just 72 hours after the parade, all 31 hospitals in Philadelphia were complete, and by the end of the week, 2600 people were dead.

George Dehner, writer of Global Flu and You: A History of Influenza, says that while Krusen's decision to hold the parade was certainly a "bad idea," the rate of infection in Philadelphia already rose to an end in September.

"Perhaps, the Liberty Loan parade poured gasoline on the flames," says Dehner, "but it was cooking pretty well along already."

The reaction from public health in St. Louis could not have been more different. Even before the city had confirmed the first case of Spanish flu, health commissioner Dr. Max Starkloff had local doctors on high alert and wrote an editorial in the St. Louis Post-Dispatch on the significance of avoiding crowds.

When a flu epidemic first spread into the civilian community of St. Louis at a nearby military base, Starkloff wasted no time closing the schools, shutting down movie theaters and pool halls, and banning all public gatherings. Business owners have tried to resist, but Starkloff and the mayor held their ground. When infections swelled as expected, a network of volunteer nurses treated thousands of sick people at home.

Dehner says public health authorities in St. Louis could "flatten the curve" and prevent the flu outbreak from spreading overnight as it did in Philadelphia because of those precautions.

"In such a short period, it's that crush of new cases that fully overwhelm the sufficiency of a community," says Dehner. "That magnifies any issues you already have."

The peak mortality rate in St. Louis was just one-eighth of the death rate in Philadelphia at its highest, according to a 2007 study of The Spanish flu death reports. That is not to say St. Louis survived the outbreak unharmed. Dehner says The Spanish flu's third outbreak, which returned in the late winter and spring of 1919, struck the midwestern city especially hard.

Health officials in San Francisco put their complete confidence behind the gauze masks. Governor of California William Stephens proclaimed it was the "patriotic duty of every American citizen" to wear a mask, and finally, San Francisco made it the rule. People found without a mask or inappropriately wearing it in public were arrested, charged with "disturbing the peace" and fined $5.

In his book, Barry says that the gauze masks reported by city officials were "99 percent proof against influenza" were hardly successful at all. The relatively low infection rates of San Francisco in October were possibly due to well-organized campaigns to quarantine all naval facilities prior to the outbreak of the flu, plus early attempts to close schools, ban social gatherings, and close all places of "public amusement."

A whistle blast on November 21 indicated that San Franciscans were finally able to take off their masks, and the San Francisco Chronicle identified "sidewalks and runnels ... strewn with the remnants of a tortuous month."

But when the third wave of Spanish flu struck in January 1919, San Francisco's luck ran out. Believing masks were what first rescued them, companies and theater owners fought back against the public orders. As a result, San Francisco ended up having some of the highest Spanish flu death rates nationally. The 2007 report showed that it could have decreased deaths by 90 percent if San Francisco had maintained all of its anti-flu protections in place through the spring of 1919.

THE VACCINE DEVELOPMENT

In 1918 The Spanish flu was dubbed an outbreak that killed at least 50 million people. Since then, what have we learned?

Another threat to human life was looming in autumn 1918, at the end of World War I. While the danger had risen since the previous year, The Spanish flu has reached pandemic levels. The disease spread across Earth almost everywhere, including the Arctic. However, the Spanish press was amongst the first to report the case in-depth at the end of World War I, and the Spanish king was himself infected, leading to the erroneous impression that the disease originated in Spain.

Once government leaders understood the risk, cities took aggressive steps to stop the disease from spreading. Schools, theaters, and other public meeting places were forced to close, and an enormous amount of money was allocated by the United States government to stop the spread. Governments created and encouraged vaccines, but we now know they were targeting the wrong strain of influenza. Ultimately, it is reported that between 50 and 100 million people died from the disease or disease complications.

While attempts at vaccination were made during the pandemic, in the 1940s, the functional version of flu vaccines began in the United States. Thomas Francis Jr. and Jonas Salk were influential in creating flu vaccines and were later best known for their work on the polio vaccine. In 1945, during World War II, the first authorized version of the vaccine was given to the troops. The next year all people were able to get vaccinated.

Influenza viruses can mutate through antigenic drift and change, which requires the constant adaptation of varieties of vaccines. Since introducing new guidelines in 1973, the World Health Organization (WHO) has identified the three most likely influenza strains, or candidate vaccine viruses (CVVs), to be used in the flu shot that year. There are also quadrivalent vaccines on the market.

Up to recently, nearly all flu vaccines were made using fertilized chicken eggs to spread the virus. This technique includes the growth in separate eggs of each of the three predicted CVVs and the fusion of the three into one. One of this approach's key benefits is that the eggs are cheaper and spread to high titers influenza. But there are also disadvantages. The egg-based vaccines have triggered allergic reactions in several unusual instances. Suppose an avian influenza strain was to become virulent. In that case, it could decimate poultry populations and cause a shortage of eggs for consumption or manufacture of vaccines that occurred with the highly pathogenic H5N2 during 2015. Viral vector vaccines are now on the market, which can be beneficial to the poultry producers if another H5 outbreak like this occurs. Those vaccines use the Same Pathogen Free (SPF) cells or eggs from Charles River.

Nevertheless, egg-based strategies can be time-consuming and volatile, with six months between

CVV isolation and finished vaccines, and variations in the amount of vaccine each egg harvests. Hence producers of influenza vaccines are searching for alternatives.

As an alternative, researchers focused on cell-based vaccines to replace the traditional form of eggs. In 2016, The Food and Drug Administration (FDA) had approved the development of Novartis' vaccine, Flucelvax, using cell-based virus isolation. In this method, cultured animal cells are used instead of eggs to incubate the viruses. This process not only removes the potential problem of an influenza outbreak but also allows for faster development, although not generally faster than conventional methods in which influenza in eggs incubates within 48-72 hours.

There have been five more influenza pandemics since The Spanish flu outbreak, most recently in 2009. Thankfully, with the advent of vaccines and other modern health care developments, none were quite as lethal as the pandemic of 1918. Lacking a universal flu vaccine, though, and with certain individuals unable to get an annual shot, it's only a matter of time before another outbreak. Influenza is a troublesome virus, and this year has also made headlines, with new strains found in dogs. But with science increasingly evolving, such as cell-based vaccines, future physicians are ready to battle the flu.

CHAPTER 6

LESSONS TO REMEMBER FROM THE GREAT INFLUENZA 1918 -1920

When we are still struggling with a pandemic, it's hard to think about how to deal with urgent social issues like systemic racism and inequality. Some of us make decisions to protest in large groups by weighing the risk of catching the new virus and spreading it to our family against the urgent need to change the way we think about race in that country.

When it suits us, pandemics do not strike. We were fighting World War I in March 1918 when the first cases of pandemic flu were reported. So, people were busy back then too.

During the flu pandemic of 1918, about 500 million people - around a third of the world's population at the time - were infected with flu. It left 50 million people dead. There was no vaccine back then. There were no effective remedies - neither for the flu nor for bacterial pneumonia that followed. Health care services around the country were utterly overloaded, and patients could not get the treatment they wanted.

There are major variations between today's pandemic and 1918 one. For instance, an influenza virus caused the 1918 flu pandemic, and a virus from Coronaviridae triggers the actual one. And then, the world was a different place, with much slower travel options, fewer people, but more crowding in many locations.

Yet the flu pandemic of 1918 taught us valuable lessons that still resonate today. Here they are :

1. Trusted tools work.

No World Health Organization existed in 1918, and there were no US Centers for Disease Control and Prevention. Each town reacted by itself to the pandemic. Cities have taken measures by counting the number of people who have had flu, by isolating and quarantining sick families, by shutting theaters and public transit, by ordering masks in public. Sounds familiar?

When cities were able to apply certain methods systematically, the curve was flattened. The more people got ill as they strayed from these methods.

2. Pandemics are not fair.

Today, the actual pandemic highlights differences between people with various forms of privilege in health and healthcare experience. Similarly, not all people were affected equally in 1918. People who had chronic health problems had a greater risk of dying. In reality, soldiers and people living in poverty and crowded conditions were more likely to become ill. Pandemics occur in all corners of the world. Everyone, each society needs the ability to be safe and able to stop the spread.

3. We cannot do this alone.

We respect our freedom, but we are taught by pandemics how interdependent we really are. We aren't the only ones affecting our health. It's

The Spanish Flu

important to your health, whether I wear a mask. If I plan to go out in public with a bit of cough, your health is affected. You may need hospital treatment, but if we haven't all done our part to stop the virus's spreading, you may not have room for that. I might not be able to get the preventive care I need if my employer does not have quality health insurance. The Flu of 1918 illustrated how we are all connected. Many nations responded after the pandemic by supplying guaranteed health coverage to all their citizens. Like the new virus, the flu did not honor any city, state, or national frontier. The International Bureau for Fighting Epidemics, a forerunner of WHO, was established in 1919.

Some scholars have noted that we avoided learning about the pandemic of 1918 overtime, and some of those lessons have been overlooked. They are valuable lessons, however, and we are relearning them. But let's make sure we remember this time.

CHAPTER 7

SIMILARITIES AND COMPARISON WITH THE ACTUAL WORLD PANDEMIC

As the 21st-century world struggles to rein in the actual pandemic, many public health authorities are looking out for insights into past pandemics that may help reduce and alleviate this epidemic. While there have been many pandemics, including Black Death, HIV, and cholera, historians most often cited the 1918 Spanish flu pandemic.

There are many parallels between the current pandemic and the one that started in 1918, but the magnitude of the crises was different. To date, the actual pandemic has killed more than 100,000 people in the US and more than 350,000 worldwide. While this is a staggering number of

The Spanish Flu

deaths, compared with the 40 million who died during the Spanish influenza pandemic, it pales.

The reasons behind these two pandemics

A study on the existence of the new virus, which is the cause of our current health epidemic, is still ongoing. Still, there are some details most virologists agree on regarding the existence of it.

- Like other viruses, the one that triggers the SARS-CoV-2 mark it can adapt to target new species. SARS-CoV-2 has been theorized as originating in bats and spreading to humans.

- SARS-CoV-2 is much more dangerous than previously found viruses from the Coronaviridae family because it attacks human cells so readily, especially those in the throat and lungs.

- With more than 30,000 genetic bases, SARS-CoV-2 is incredibly large, making it three times the size of HIV or hepatitis C and twice the influenza size. This enormous genetic diversity can allow it to recombine faster with other SARS-CoV-2 strains and grow into more problematic ones.

- In contrast to many other viruses, SARS-CoV-2 also has a gene-reading system that prevents mutations. This is possibly why antiviral drugs are less effective against SARS-CoV-2 because such drugs trigger mutations that reduce the virus's lethality.

- While The Spanish flu pandemic hit more than a century ago, its genetic structure and morphology were not discovered until recently by scientists. Researchers also discovered new knowledge of the virus using the frozen DNA of an Inuit woman who died from Spanish flu.

- This influenza strain is known as H1N1 and originated in birds. The 1918 strain had only recently spread to humans, resulting in fewer people having immunity, and the virus was especially lethal compared to more viable older viruses.

- Influenza typically triggers globe-wide epidemics with a mortality rate of around 0.1%, but this Spanish flu had a mortality rate of 2.5%. This strain's precise virulence is not yet fully known, but most researchers accept that several genetic factors have contributed.

- A highly significant aspect of the Spanish influenza virus was its ability to replicate rapidly and linger in the lungs. One analysis of mice showed that the H1N1 virus was 39,000 times higher in mice lungs than other kinds of influenza.

Similarities between SARS-CoV-2 and the Spanish flu

We are still amid the new pandemic, so it's hard to predict the nature and after-effects of this public health epidemic. Still, there are already some striking parallels with the 1918 pandemic. Both the SARS-CoV-2 and the H1N1 viruses were unique to human populations, meaning they did not have natural immunity. This explains in part why the fatality rates for both diseases were far higher than outbreaks of seasonal influenza.

Like the current pandemic, the flu of 1918 had several waves - although the current situation is still evolving, future pandemics are likely to be mimicable. The pandemic of 1918 emerged in the US, Europe, and Asia almost simultaneously until it spread through the global population. In the spring of 1918, this initial wave was mild, with most people recovering from the infection.

In the fall of the same year, a second wave erupted but with even more lethality. A number of the infected this time died within hours or days, rather than recovering. The most frequent cause of death has been fluid that filled the lungs due to secondary infections such as pneumonia.

Many researchers suggest the actual pandemic has a similar working mechanism on patients. Like the flu of 1918, SARS-CoV-2 induces a huge release of immune proteins called cytokines. This "cytokine storm" affects mainly the lung tissue that dies as a result. The resulting condition frequently includes pneumonia accompanied by a lack of oxygen and eventually death.

CONCLUSION

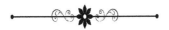

In a mere eight months, a previously unknown virus has brought the planet to its knees. Yet today's pandemic won't be the last one, or maybe even the worst.

It is estimated that an average of 650,000 to 840,000 unknown viral species lurk in wildlife to infect humans. In time, population development, climate change, urbanization, globalization, the ongoing degradation of wildlife habitats, and wild species' harvesting have taken these viruses closer to humans than ever before.

Pandemics may become the new normal.

But that does not have to be the case. Pandemics are preventable, and there are three important things the world should do to prevent them.

First, we might be able to build a global early warning system. Much like earthquakes and tsunami, an early warning system could allow early detection and fast response to an outbreak before it spreads. It will gather information through a combination of artificial intelligence (AI) surveillance, zoonotic reconnaissance, and investigation of outbreaks.

Pandemics typically begin when a virus or other pathogen hops from animals to humans, also called a zoonotic spillover. The viruses that triggered Middle East respiratory syndrome (MERS), severe acute respiratory syndrome (SARS), and now SARS-CoV-2 pandemics all jumped from bats to humans through an intermediary animal host: for SARS, it was civets, for MERS, it was camels and a still unknown intermediary for the actual one. Routine connection identification between these sentinel animals and the people in close contact with them may provide early notice of an imminent outbreak.

Searching across the globe for the possible connections is pointless unless you know where to look. AI can help.

Scientists have identified global geographic hotspots that are most vulnerable to zoonotic spillovers using machine learning algorithms to sift through molecular, ecological, epidemiologic, and climate data.

Second, by improving public health, we will avoid potential pandemics. If local, national, and global public health networks can not mount an efficient response to an outbreak, early alerts will be useless. Places in the world that have flattened the epidemic curve so far- such as South Korea, Taiwan, and Singapore - all have strong public health systems that have taken early action, developed a centralized command, implemented an organized and science-based strategy, mobilized vast technical and human resources, ramped up testing and constant monitoring, and provided trustworthy and accessible information to the public

By comparison, monitoring appears to be insufficient in the United States, and persistent underfunding has left the most state and local public health departments without sufficient resources to monitor mass contacts. Tragically, the federal government was incompetent, naive, and disorganized in its reaction, despite plenty of early warnings, leaving the states to fend for themselves. The new pandemic highlights the shortcomings of public health programs in the US and worldwide, which need to be resolved before the next pandemic.

Third, by mitigating the possibility of spillovers, we can avoid potential pandemics at the root. The preservation of natural habitats from unrelenting human invasion and the establishment of buffer zones around protected areas are important long-term priorities. More urgently, we should stop the trade in wildlife, not only by restricting, controlling, or closing down live animal markets like those in Wuhan but also by implementing international law to tackle illicit and unsustainable trade in wildlife. The US and China, respectively, are responsible for 60% of global

Made in the USA
Middletown, DE
12 December 2020

27414160R00076